KETO COOK
BEGIN1

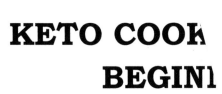

The Ultimate Keto Diet Cookbook for Beginners with Healthy and Mouthwatering Recipes to Boost Your Metabolism and Burn Fat Quickly

Written by

Sam Gallo

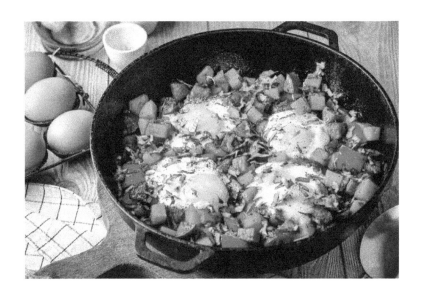

© Copyright 2021 all rights reserved

This report is towards furnishing precise and reliable data concerning the point and issue secured. It was conceivable that the manufacturer was not required to do bookkeeping, legally approved, or anything else, competent administrations. If the exhortation is relevant, valid, or qualified, a rehearsed person should be requested during the call.

It is not appropriate to reproduce, copy, or distribute any portion of this report in either electronic methods or in the community written. Recording this delivery is carefully disclaimed, and the ability of this report is not permitted until the distributor has written a license. All rights. All rights held.

The data provided in this document is expressed in an honest and predictable way, like any risk, in so far as abstention or anything else, is a singular and articulate duty for the beneficiary per user to use or mistreat any approaches, procedures or bearing contained within it. No legal responsibility or blame shall be held against the distributor for any reparation, loss, or money-related misfortune because of the results, whether explicitly or implied.

All copyrights not held by the distributor are asserted by individual authors.

Table of Contents

INTRODUCTION 9

BREAKFAST RECIPES.. 10

COCONUT BLINI WITH BERRY DRIZZLE 12

PESTO BREAD TWISTS 14

BROCCOLI HASH BROWNS 15

SPINACH & FONTINA CHEESE NEST BITES 16

MIXED SEED BREAD 17

BREAKFAST EGG MUFFINS WITH BACON........................... 19

CHORIZO & AVOCADO EGGS 20

SWISS CHEESE CHORIZO WAFFLES 21

STARTER AND SALAD.. 22

ALMOND BREAD & BACON PUDDING.................................... 23

ONE-PAN MIXED GARDEN GREENS 24

WALNUT BROCCOLI "RICE".. 25

MACKEREL AND GREEN BEANS SALAD................................ 26

CHICKEN & BOK CHOY CAESAR SALAD 27

SHRIMP SALAD WITH CAULIFLOWER & CUCUMBER 28

ITALIAN TRICOLORE SALAD 29

SOUP AND STEWS.. 30

TOFU GOULASH SOUP 31

ROSEMARY ONION SOUP.. 32

GINGER-SPINACH EGG BENEDICT SOUP 33

TOMATO SOUP WITH PARMESAN CROUTONS 34

POWER GREEN SOUP 36

LUNCH AND DINNER... 37

KALE & MUSHROOM GALETTE.. 38

BRAISED SAGE-FLAVORED LAMB CHOPS 40

TURNIP CHIPS WITH AVOCADO DIP 41

BURRITOS WITH AVOCADO GREEK YOGURT FILLING 42

CHEESY STUFFED VENISON TENDERLOIN 43

PROSCIUTTO EGGPLANT BOATS 44

CHEESY MUSHROOM PIE 45

SPINACH & CHEESE FLANK STEAK PINWHEELS 47

PROSCIUTTO-WRAPPED CHICKEN WITH ASPARAGUS 48

MUSHROOM BROCCOLI FAUX RISOTTO................................. 49

POULTRY 50

WORCESTERSHIRE CHICKEN PEANUT PUFFS....................... 51

CHARGRILLED CHILI CHICKEN 52

CREAMY CHICKEN WITH MUSHROOMS.................................. 53

CHICKEN THIGHS WITH GREENS 54

BAKED CHEESE CHICKEN WITH ACORN SQUASH 55

CHICKEN & VEGETABLE BAKE... 56

CHEESE-CRUSTED CHICKEN BREASTS 57

CREAMY CHICKEN THIGHS WITH CAPERS............................ 58

ROSEMARY CHICKEN& PUMPKIN BAKE 59

BEEF 60

BEEF TACO PIZZA 61

BEEF WITH CAULI RICE & CASHEW NUTS............................ 62

EASY PRESSURE-COOKED SHREDDED BEEF 63

MUSHROOM & BELL PEPPER BEEF SKEWERS 64

BEEF & SHIITAKE MUSHROOM STIR-FRY 65

COCONUT BEEF WITH MUSHROOM & OLIVE SAUCE............. 66

MAPLE BBQ RIB STEAK... 67

SMOKED PAPRIKA GRILLED RIBS...................................... 68

PORK... 69

SLOW COOKER PULLED PORK 70

TASTY PORK CHOPS WITH CAULIFLOWER STEAKS............. 72

LEMONY GREEK PORK TENDERLOIN 73

MUSHROOM PORK MEATBALLS WITH PARSNIPS.................. 74

SPICY GRILLED PORK SPARERIBS 75

SESAME PORK MEATBALLS 77

PORK BELLY WITH CREAMY COCONUT KALE....................... 78

FLAVORFUL CHIPOTLE-COFFEE PORK CHOPS 79

SEAFOOD 80

MAHI MAHI WITH DILL SOUR CREAM TOPPING 81

MEDITERRANEAN TILAPIA 82

SPEEDY TILAPIA TACOS... 83

COD FRITTERS WITH AVOCADO SALSA 84

VEGAN AND VEGETARIAN 85

STUFFED PORTOBELLO MUSHROOMS 86

CHEESY ROASTED VEGETABLE SPAGHETTI 87

VEGETARIAN KETOGENIC BURGERS 88

TEMPEH TACO CUPS 89

RICH VEGGIE PASTA PRIMAVERA 90

MUSHROOM WHITE PIZZA.. 92

CHEESY BROCCOLI NACHOS WITH SALSA 93

SNACKS AND SIDE DISH... 95

CHILI BAKED ZUCCHINI STICKS WITH AIOLI 96

CAULIFLOWER RICE & BACON GRATIN 97

DELICIOUS PANCETTA STRAWBERRIES............................... 98

CREAMY HAM & PARSNIP PUREE.. 99

ROASTED HAM WITH RADISHES 100

ROSEMARY CHEESE CHIPS WITH GUACAMOLE 101

CHIVE & GREEN BEAN HAM ROLLS 102

DESSERT.. 103

COCONUT BUTTER ICE CREAM 104

CHIA PUDDING 105

MOM'S WALNUT COOKIES.. 106

ALMOND ICE CREAM.. 107

DARK CHOCOLATE CHEESECAKE BITES 108

CARDAMOM COOKIES 109

CHOCOLATE ICE BOMBS.. 110

Introduction

Want to follow a ketogenic diet but not sure where to start? Struggling with finding delicious and tummy-filling recipes when going "against the grains"? Do not worry! In this book you will find mouth-watering delights for any occasion and any eater, you will not believe that these recipes will help you restore your health and slim down your body.

Successfully practiced for more than nine decades, the ketogenic diet hs proven to be the ultimate long-term diet for any person. The restriction list may frighten many, but the truth is, this diet is super adaptable, and the food combinations and tasty meals are pretty endless.

Most people believe that our bodies are designed to run on carbohydrates. We think that ingesting carbohydrates is the only way to provide our bodies with the energy they need to function normally. However, what many people don't know is that carbohydrates are not the only source of fuel our bodies can use. Our bodies can also use fat as an energy source! When we decide to ditch carbs and provide our bodies with more fat, then we've begun our journey into the ketogenic diet, and this cookbook will be the guide you need to make your journey simple and enjoyable...let's start!

Breakfast recipes

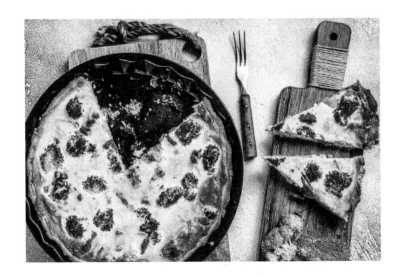

Coconut Blini with Berry Drizzle

Ingredients for 6 servings

Pancakes
1 cup cream cheese
1 cup coconut flour
1 tsp salt
2 tsp xylitol
1 tsp baking soda
1 tsp baking powder
1 ½ cups coconut milk
1 tsp vanilla extract
6 large eggs
¼ cup olive oil

Blackberry Sauce
3 cups fresh blackberries
1 lemon, juiced
½ cup xylitol
½ tsp arrowroot starch
A pinch of salt

Directions and Total Time: approx. 40 minutes

Put coconut flour, salt, xylitol, baking soda and powder in a bowl and whisk to combine. Add in milk, cream cheese, vanilla, eggs, and olive oil and whisk until smooth. Set a pan and pour in a small ladle of batter. Cook on one side for 2 minutes, flip, and cook for 2 minutes. Transfer to a plate and repeat the cooking process until the batter is exhausted. Pour the berries and half cup of water into a saucepan and bring to a boil. Simmer for 12 minutes. Pour in xylitol, stir, and continue cooking for 5 minutes. Stir in salt and lemon juice. Mix arrowroot starch with 1 tbsp of water; pour the mixture into the berries. Stir and continue cooking the sauce until it thickens. Serve.

Per serving: Cal 433; Net Carbs 4.9g; Fat 39g; Protein 8.2g

Pesto Bread Twists

Ingredients for 6 servings

1 tbsp flax seed powder + 3 tbsp water
1½ cups grated mozzarella
4 tbsp coconut flour
½ cup almond flour
1 tsp baking powder
5 tbsp butter
2 oz pesto

Directions and Total Time: approx. 35 minutes

For flax egg, mix flax seed powder with water in a bowl, and let to soak for 5 minutes. Preheat oven to 350 F. Line a baking sheet with parchment paper. In a bowl, combine coconut flour, almond flour, and baking powder. Melt butter and cheese in a skillet and stir in the flax egg. Mix in flour mixture until a firm dough forms. Divide the mixture between 2 parchment papers, then use a rolling pin to flatten out the dough of about an inch's thickness. Remove the parchment paper on top and spread pesto all over the dough. Cut the dough into strips, twist each piece, and place on the baking sheet. Brush with olive oil and bake for 15-20 minutes until golden brown.

Per serving: Cal 206; Net Carbs 3g; Fat 17g; Protein 8g

Broccoli Hash Browns

Ingredients for 4 servings

3 tbsp flax seed powder + 9 tbsp water
1 head broccoli, rinsed and cut into florets
½ white onion, grated
5 tbsp vegan butter

Directions and Total Time: approx. 35 minutes

In a bowl, mix flax seed powder with water and allow soaking for 5 minutes. Pour broccoli into a food processor and pulse until smoothly grated. Transfer to a bowl, add in flax egg and onion. Mix and let sit for 10 minutes to firm up a bit. Melt butter in a skillet. Ladle scoops of the broccoli mixture into the skillet, flatten and fry until golden brown, 8 minutes, turning once. Transfer the hash browns to a plate and repeat the frying process for the remaining broccoli mixture. Serve warm.

Per serving: Cal 287; Net Carbs 4g; Fat 25g; Protein 8g

Spinach & Fontina Cheese Nest Bites

Ingredients for 4 servings

4 tbsp shredded Pecorino Romano cheese
2 tbsp shredded fontina
1 tbsp olive oil
1 clove garlic, grated
½ lb spinach, chopped
4 eggs
Salt and black pepper to taste

Directions and Total Time: approx. 40 minutes

Preheat oven to 350 F. Warm oil in a skillet, add garlic, and sauté for 2 minutes. Add in spinach to wilt about 5 minutes and season with salt and pepper. Stir in 2 tbsp of Pecorino Romano cheese and fontina cheese and remove from the heat. Allow cooling. Mold 4 (firm separate) spinach nests on a greased sheet and crack an egg into each nest. Sprinkle with the remaining Pecorino Romano cheese. Bake for 15 minutes. Serve right away.

Per serving: Cal 230; Net Carbs 4g; Fat 17.5g; Protein 12g

Mixed Seed Bread

Ingredients for 6 servings

3 tbsp ground flax seeds
¾ cup coconut flour
1 cup almond flour
3 tsp baking powder
5 tbsp sesame seeds
½ cup chia seeds
1 tsp ground caraway seeds
1 tsp hemp seeds
¼ cup psyllium husk powder
1 tsp salt
1 cup vegan cream cheese
½ cup melted coconut oil
¾ cup coconut cream
1 tbsp poppy seeds

Directions and Total Time: approx. 55 minutes

Preheat oven to 350 F. Line a loaf pan with parchment paper. For flax egg, whisk flax seed powder with ½ cup water and let the mixture soak for 5 minutes. In a bowl, combine coconut and almond flours, baking powder, sesame, chia, caraway and hemp seeds, psyllium husk powder, and salt. Whisk cream cheese, oil, cream, and flax egg in another bowl.

Pour the liquid ingredients into the dry ingredients, and continue whisking until a dough forms. Transfer to loaf pan, sprinkle with poppy seeds, and bake for 45 minutes. Remove parchment paper with the bread and allow cooling on a rack. Slice and serve.

Per serving: Cal 230; Net Carbs 3g; Fat 19g; Protein 7g

Breakfast Egg Muffins with Bacon

Ingredients for 6 servings

12 eggs
¼ cup coconut milk
Salt and black pepper to taste
1 cup Colby cheese, grated
12 slices bacon
4 jalapeño peppers, minced

Directions and Total Time: approx. 30 minutes

Preheat oven to 370 F. Crack the eggs into a bowl and whisk with coconut milk until combined. Season with salt and pepper and stir in the colby cheese. Line each hole of a muffin tin with a slice of bacon and fill each with the egg mixture two-thirds way up. Top with the jalapeños and bake in the oven for 18-20 minutes or until puffed and golden. Remove, let cool for a few minutes, and serve.

Per serving: Cal 302; Net Carbs 3.2g; Fat 2g; Protein 20g

Chorizo & Avocado Eggs

Ingredients for 4 servings

2 tbsp ghee
1 yellow onion, sliced
4 oz chorizo, sliced
1 cup chopped collard greens
1 avocado, chopped
4 eggs

Directions and Total Time: approx. 25 minutes

Preheat oven to 370 F. Melt ghee in a pan and sauté onion for 2 minutes. Add in chorizo and cook for 2 more minutes, stirring often. Introduce the collard greens with a splash of water to wilt, season with salt, stir, and cook for 3 minutes. Mix in avocado and turn the heat off. Create four holes in the mixture and crack the eggs into each hole. Sprinkle with salt and pepper and slide the pan into the preheated oven. Bake for 6 minutes. Serve right away.

Per serving: Cal 274; Net Carbs 4g; Fat 23g; Protein 13g

Swiss Cheese Chorizo Waffles

Ingredients for 6 servings

3 chorizo sausages, cooked, chopped
1 cup Gruyere cheese, shredded
6 eggs
6 tbsp coconut milk
1 tsp Spanish spice mix
Salt and black pepper, to taste

Directions and Total Time: approx. 30 minutes

In a bowl, beat the eggs, Spanish spice mix, black pepper, salt, and coconut milk. Add in the Gruyere cheese and chopped sausages. Grease the waffle iron with cooking spray. Working in batches, cook the dough for 5 minutes.

Per serving: Cal 316; Net Carbs: 2g; Fat: 25g; Protein: 20g

Starter and Salad

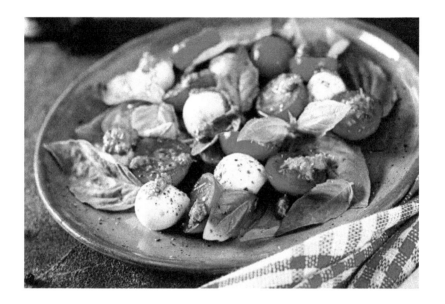

Almond Bread & Bacon Pudding

Ingredients for 4 servings

1 tbsp olive oil
3 bacon slices, chopped
1 orange bell pepper, chopped
3 tbsp butter, softened
6 slices low carb bread
1 red onion, finely chopped
3 eggs
1 ½ cup almond milk
3 tbsp grated cheddar cheese
2 tbsp grated Parmesan

Directions and Total Time: approx. 35 minutes

Preheat oven to 300 F. Heat oil in a skillet and add the bacon and bell pepper. Cook until the bacon browns. Brush a baking dish with the butter and apply some on both sides of each bread slice. Cut into cubes and arrange in the baking dish. Scatter with onions, bacon, and bell pepper. In a bowl, beat eggs with almond milk and pour the mixture over. Sprinkle with cheddar and Parmesan cheeses and bake for 20 minutes until golden. Serve warm.

Per serving: Cal 362; Net Carbs 7.7g; Fat 27g; Protein 13g

One-Pan Mixed Garden Greens

Ingredients for 4 servings

2 shallots, finely sliced
1 tsp swerve sugar
2 tbsp red wine vinegar
2 tbsp butter
1 tsp cumin powder
1 garlic clove, minced
1 cup asparagus, chopped
2 cups mixed garden greens
4 tbsp chopped parsley
1 tbsp olive oil
2 tbsp pine nuts

Directions and Total Time: approx. 25 minutes

In a bowl, whisk shallots, swerve sugar, and vinegar and set aside. Melt butter in a skillet and stir in cumin and garlic for 1 minute. Add in asparagus to soften for 5 minutes. Mix in mixed greens. Reduce the heat to low and steam the vegetables for 1 minute. Stir in parsley. Drizzle with olive oil and garnish with pine nuts to serve.

Per serving: Cal 79; Net Carbs 3.5g; Fat 6.1g; Protein 1.9g

Walnut Broccoli "Rice"

Ingredients for 4 servings

2 tbsp butter
1 garlic clove, minced
2 heads large broccoli, riced
½ cup vegetable broth
Salt and black pepper to taste
¼ cup toasted walnuts, chopped
4 tbsp sesame seeds, toasted
2 tbsp chopped cilantro

Directions and Total Time: approx. 25 minutes

Melt butter in a pot and stir in garlic. Cook until fragrant, for 1 minute and addi in broccoli and vegetable broth. Allow steaming for 2 minutes. Season with salt and pepper and cook for 3-5 minutes. Pour in walnuts, sesame seeds, and cilantro. Fluff the rice and serve warm.

Per serving: Cal 240; Net Carbs 3g; Fat 15g; Protein 11g

Mackerel and Green Beans Salad

Ingredients for 2 servings

2 mackerel fillets
2 hard-boiled eggs, sliced
1 tbsp coconut oil
2 cups green beans
1 avocado, sliced
4 cups mixed salad greens
2 tbsp olive oil
2 tbsp lemon juice
1 tsp Dijon mustard
Salt and black pepper to taste

Directions and Total Time: approx. 25 minutes

Fill a saucepan with water and add the beans and salt. Cook over medium heat for 3 minutes. Drain and set aside. Melt the coconut oil in a pan over medium heat. Add the mackerel fillets and cook for about 4 minutes per side, or until opaque and crispy. Divide the greens between two salad bowls. Top with mackerel, egg and avocado slices. In a separate bowl, whisk together lemon juice, olive oil, mustard, salt, and pepper and drizzle over the salad. Serve.

Per serving: Cal 525; Net Carbs 7.6g; Fat 42g; Protein 27g

Chicken & Bok Choy Caesar Salad

Ingredients for 4 servings

4 boneless and skinless chicken thighs
¼ cup lemon juice
4 tbsp olive oil
½ cup Caesar salad dressing
12 bok choy, cut lengthwise
2 tbsp shaved Parmesan

Directions and Total Time: approx. 1 hour 20 minutes

Combine the chicken thighs, lemon juice, and 2 tbsp olive oil in a Ziploc bag. Seal the bag, shake to combine, and refrigerate for 1 hour. Preheat grill to medium heat and grill the chicken for 4 minutes per side. Brush bok choy with the remaining olive oil and grill for 3 minutes. Remove to a serving platter. Top with the chicken and drizzle the Caesar dressing over. Sprinkle with Parmesan.

Per serving: Cal 529; Net Carbs 5g; Fat 39g; Protein 33g

Shrimp Salad with Cauliflower & Cucumber

Ingredients for 6 servings

1 cauliflower head, florets only
1 lb medium shrimp
3 tbsp olive oil
2 cucumber, chopped
3 tbsp chopped dill
¼ cup lemon juice
2 tbsp lemon zest

Directions and Total Time: approx. 30 minutes

Heat 1 tbsp olive oil in a skillet and cook the shrimp until opaque, about 10 minutes. Microwave cauliflower florets for 5 minutes. Place shrimp, cauliflower, and cucumber in a large bowl. Whisk together the remaining olive oil, lemon zest, lemon juice, and dill in another bowl. Pour the dressing over and toss to combine. Serve.

Per serving: Cal 214; Net Carbs 5g; Fat 17g; Protein 15g

Italian Tricolore Salad

Ingredients for 4 servings

¼ lv buffalo mozzarella cheese, sliced
3 tomatoes, sliced
1 avocado, sliced
8 black olives
2 tbsp pesto sauce
2 tbsp olive oil

Directions and Total Time: approx. 10 minutes

Arrange the tomato slices on a serving platter. Place the avocado slices in the middle. Arrange the olives around the avocado slices. Drop slices of mozzarella on the platter. Drizzle pesto sauce and olive oil all over and serve.

Per serving: Cal 290; Net Carbs 4.3g; Fat 25g; Protein 9g

Soup and stews

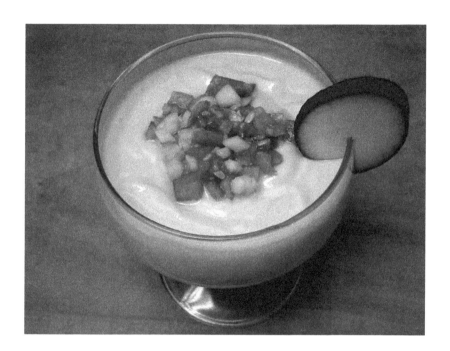

Tofu Goulash Soup

Ingredients for 4 servings

8 oz chopped butternut squash
1 ½ cups tofu, crumbled
3 tbsp butter
1 white onion, chopped
2 garlic cloves, minced
1 red bell pepper
1 tbsp paprika powder
¼ tsp red chili flakes
Salt and black pepper to taste
1 ½ cups crushed tomatoes
3 cups vegetable broth
1 ½ tsp red wine vinegar
Chopped cilantro to serve

Directions and Total Time: approx. 25 minutes

Melt butter in a pot set over medium heat and sauté onion and garlic for 3 minutes until fragrant and soft. Stir in tofu and cook for 3 minutes. Add in butternut squash, bell pepper, paprika, red chili flakes, salt, and pepper. Cook for 2 minutes. Pour in tomatoes and vegetable broth. Bring to a boil, then reduce the heat to simmer for 10 minutes; mix in vinegar. Garnish with cilantro and serve.

Per serving: Cal 481; Fat 41.8g; Net Carbs 9g; Protein 12g

Rosemary Onion Soup

Ingredients for 4 servings

2 tbsp butter
1 tbsp olive oil
3 sliced white onions
2 garlic cloves, thinly sliced
2 tsp almond flour
½ cup dry white wine
2 sprigs chopped rosemary
Salt and black pepper to taste
2 cups almond milk
1 cup grated Parmesan cheese

Directions and Total Time: approx. 35 minutes

Heat butter and olive oil in a pot over medium heat and sauté onions and garlic for 6-7 minutes. Reduce the heat to low and cook further for 10 minutes. Stir in almond flour, white wine, salt, pepper, and rosemary and pour in 2 cups water. Bring to a boil and simmer for 10 minutes. Pour in almond milk and half of the Parmesan cheese. Stir to melt the cheese and spoon into a serving bowl. Top with the remaining Parmesan cheese and serve.

Per serving: Cal 340; Net Carbs 5.6g; Fat 23g, Protein 15g

Ginger-Spinach Egg Benedict Soup

Ingredients for 4 servings

2 tbsp butter
1 tbsp sesame oil
1 small onion, finely sliced
3 garlic cloves, minced
2 tsp ginger paste
2 cups baby spinach, chopped
2 cups chopped green beans
4 cups vegetable stock
3 tbsp chopped cilantro
4 eggs

Directions and Total Time: approx. 35 minutes

Melt butter in a pot and sauté onion, garlic, and ginger for 4 minutes, stirring frequently. Stir in spinach, allowing wilting, and pour in green beans and vegetable stock. Bring to boil and simmer for 10 minutes. Transfer the soup to a blender and puree until smooth. Bring 3 cups of vinegared water to simmer and when hot, slide in an egg to poach for 3 minutes; remove with a perforated spoon. Repeat the process with the remaining eggs, one at time. Divide the soup between 4 bowls and place an egg on each one, drizzle with sesame oil and cilantro, and serve.

Per serving: Cal 463; Net Carbs 5.8g; Fat 30g, Protein 23g

Tomato Soup with Parmesan Croutons

Ingredients for 6 servings

Parmesan Croutons:
3 egg whites
1 ¼ cups almond flour
2 tsp baking powder
5 tbsp psyllium husk powder
4 tbsp butter
4 tbsp grated Parmesan

Tomato Soup
2 lb fresh ripe tomatoes
4 cloves garlic, peeled only
1 small white onion, diced
1 red bell pepper, diced
3 tbsp olive oil
1 cup coconut cream
½ tsp dried rosemary
½ tsp dried oregano
2 tbsp chopped fresh basil
Salt and black pepper to taste

Directions and Total Time: approx. 1 hour 25 minutes

For the parmesan croutons:

Preheat oven to 350 F. Line a baking sheet with parchment paper. In a bowl, combine almond flour, baking powder, and psyllium husk powder. Mix in the egg whites and whisk for 30 seconds until well combined but not overly mixed. Form 8 flat pieces out of the dough. Place on the baking sheet while leaving enough room between each to allow rising. Bake for 30 minutes. Remove croutons to cool and break into halves. Mix butter with Parmesan cheese and spread the mixture in the inner parts of the croutons. Bake for another 5 minutes.

For the tomato soup:

In a baking dish, add tomatoes, garlic, onion, bell pepper, and drizzle with olive oil. Roast vegetables in the oven for 25 minutes and after broil for 4 minutes. Transfer to a blender and add in coconut cream, rosemary, oregano, salt, and pepper. Puree until smooth. Top with croutons.

Per serving: Cal 434; Fat 38g; Net Carbs 6g; Protein 11g

Power Green Soup

Ingredients for 4 servings

3 tbsp butter
1 cup spinach, coarsely
1 cup kale, coarsely
1 large avocado
3 ½ cups coconut cream
1 cup vegetable broth
3 tbsp chopped mint leaves
Juice from 1 lime
1 cup collard greens, chopped
3 garlic cloves, minced
3 tbsp cardamom powder
2 tbsp toasted pistachios

Directions and Total Time: approx. 15 minutes

Set a saucepan over medium heat and melt 2 tbsp of the butter. Put in spinach and kale and sauté for 5 minutes. Remove to a food processor. Add in avocado, coconut cream, vegetable broth, mint, and lime juice and puree until smooth; reserve the soup. Reheat the saucepan with the remaining butter and add in collard greens, garlic, and cardamom powder and sauté for 4 minutes. Spoon the soup into bowls and garnish with collards and pistachios.

Per serving: Cal 885; Fat 80g; Net Carbs 15g; Protein 14g

Lunch and dinner

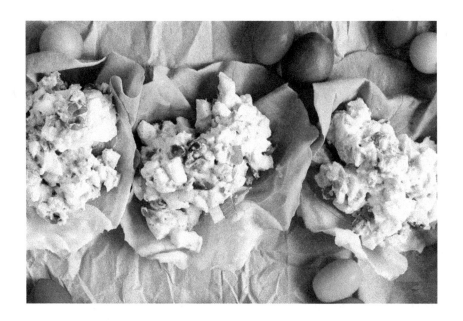

Kale & Mushroom Galette

Ingredients for 4 servings

1 tbsp flax seed powder
1 cup grated mozzarella
1 tbsp butter
½ cup almond flour
¼ cup coconut flour
½ tsp onion powder
1 tsp baking powder
3 oz cream cheese,
1 garlic clove, minced
Salt and black pepper to taste
2/3 cup kale, chopped
2 oz mushrooms, sliced
1 oz grated Parmesan
2 tbsp olive oil for brushing

Directions and Total Time: approx. 35 minutes

Preheat oven to 375 F. Line a baking sheet with parchment paper. In a bowl, mix flax seed powder with 3 tbsp water and allow sitting for 5 minutes. Place a pot over low heat, add in ½ cup mozzarella cheese and almond butter, and melt both. Turn the heat off. Stir in almond and coconut flours, onion powder, and baking powder. Pour in flax egg and combine until a quite sticky dough forms. Transfer the dough to the sheet, cover with another parchment paper and use a rolling pin to flatten into a circle.

Remove parchment paper and spread cream cheese on the dough, leaving about 2-inch border around the edges. Sprinkle with garlic, salt, and pepper. Spread kale on top of the cheese, followed by mushrooms. Sprinkle the remaining mozzarella and Parmesan cheeses on top. Fold the ends of the crust over the filling and brush with olive oil. Bake for about 25-30 minutes. Serve.

Per serving: Cal 640; Net Carbs 2g; Fat 62g; Protein 16g

Braised Sage-Flavored Lamb Chops

Ingredients for 6 servings

6 lamb chops
1 tbsp sage
1 tsp thyme
1 onion, sliced
3 garlic cloves, minced
2 tbsp olive oil
½ cup white wine
Salt and black pepper to taste

Directions and Total Time: approx. 1 hour 25 minutes

Heat the olive oil in a pan. Add onion and garlic and cook for 3 minutes, until soft; set aside. Rub sage and thyme onto the lamb and sear it in the pan for 3 minutes per side; reserve. Deglaze the pan with white wine and pour in 1 cup of water. Bring the mixture to a boil. Cook until the liquid reduces by half. Add the lamb, lower the heat, and let simmer for 1 hour. Serve warm.

Per serving: Cal 397; Net Carbs 4.3g; Fat 30g; Protein 16g

Turnip Chips with Avocado Dip

Ingredients for 6 servings

2 avocados, mashed
2 tsp lime juice
2 garlic cloves, minced
2 tbsp olive oil

For turnip chips
1 ½ pounds turnips, sliced
1 tbsp olive oil
Salt to taste
½ tsp garlic powder

Directions and Total Time: approx. 20 minutes

Stir avocado in lime juice, 2 tbsp of olive oil, and garlic until well combined. Remove to a bowl. Preheat oven to 300 F. Set turnip slices on a greased baking sheet; toss with garlic powder, 1 tbsp of olive oil, and salt. Bake for 15 minutes. Serve with chilled avocado dip.

Per serving: Cal 269; Net Carbs: 9g; Fat: 27g; Protein: 3g

Burritos with Avocado Greek Yogurt Filling

Ingredients for 4 servings

2 cups cauli rice
6 zero carb flatbread
2 cups Greek yogurt
1 ½ cups tomato herb salsa
2 avocados, sliced

Directions and Total Time: approx. 5 minutes

Pour the cauli rice in a bowl, sprinkle with water and microwave for 2 minutes.

On flatbread, spread the Greek yogurt all over and distribute the salsa on top.

Top with cauli rice and scatter the avocado evenly on top. Fold and tuck the

burritos and cut into two. Serve.

Per serving: Cal 303; Net Carbs 6g; Fat 25g; Protein 8g

Cheesy Stuffed Venison Tenderloin

Ingredients for 8 servings

2 pounds venison tenderloin
2 garlic cloves, minced
2 tbsp chopped almonds
½ cup Gorgonzola cheese
½ cup feta cheese
1 tsp chopped onion
3 tbsp olive oil

Directions and Total Time: approx. 30 minutes

Preheat oven to 360 F. Slice the tenderloin lengthwise to make a pocket for the filling. In a skillet, heat the oil and brown the meat on all sides, 8-10 minutes in total. Combine the rest of the ingredients in a bowl. Stuff the tenderloin with the filling. Shut the meat with skewers. Transfer to a baking dish along with the oil and half cup of water and cook for 25-30 minutes, until cooked through.

Per serving: Cal 194; Net Carbs 1.7g; Fat 12g; Protein 25g

Prosciutto Eggplant Boats

Ingredients for 3 servings

3 eggplants, cut into halves
1 tbsp deli mustard
2 prosciutto slices, chopped
6 eggs
Salt and black pepper to taste
¼ tsp dried parsley

Directions and Total Time: approx. 35 minutes

Scoop flesh from eggplant halves to make shells. Set the eggplant boats on a greased baking pan. Spread mustard on the bottom of every eggplant half. Split the prosciutto among eggplant boats. Crack an egg in each half, sprinkle with parsley, pepper, and salt. Set oven at 400 F. Bake for 30 minutes or until boats become tender.

Per serving: Cal 506; Net Carbs 4.5g; Fat 41g; Protein 27g

Cheesy Mushroom Pie

Ingredients for 4 servings

For the piecrust:
¼ cup butter, cold and crumbled
¼ cup almond flour
3 tbsp coconut flour
½ tsp salt
3 tbsp erythritol
1 ½ tsp vanilla extract
4 whole eggs

For the filling:
2 cups mixed mushrooms, chopped
1 cup green beans, cut into 3 pieces each
2 tbsp butter
1 yellow onion, chopped
2 garlic cloves, minced
1 green bell pepper, diced
Salt and black pepper to taste
¼ cup heavy cream
1/3 cup sour cream
½ cup almond milk
2 eggs, lightly beaten
¼ tsp nutmeg powder
1 tbsp chopped parsley
1 cup grated Monterey Jack

Directions and Total Time: approx. 2 hours

Preheat oven to 350 F. In a bowl, mix almond and coconut flours, and salt. Add in butter and mix until crumbly. Stir in erythritol and vanilla extract. Pour in the eggs one after another while mixing until formed into a ball. Flatten the dough on a clean flat surface, cover with plastic wrap, and refrigerate for 1 hour. Dust a clean flat surface with almond flour, unwrap the dough and roll out into a large rectangle. Fit into a greased pie pan and with a fork, prick the base of the crust. Bake for 15 minutes; let cool. For the filling, melt butter in a skillet over medium heat and sauté onion and garlic for 3 minutes. Add in mushrooms, bell pepper, and green beans; cook for 5 minutes. In a bowl, beat heavy cream, sour cream, almond milk, and eggs. Season with salt, pepper, and nutmeg. Stir in parsley and cheese. Spread the mushroom mixture on the baked pastry and spread the cheese filling on top. Place the pie in the oven and bake for 35 minutes. Slice and serve.

Per serving: Cal 527; Net Carbs 6.5g; Fat 43g; Protein 21g

Spinach & Cheese Flank Steak Pinwheels

Ingredients for 6 servings

1 ½ lb flank steak
Salt and black pepper to taste
1 cup ricotta cheese, crumbled
½ loose cup baby spinach
1 jalapeño pepper, chopped
¼ cup chopped basil leaves

Directions and Total Time: approx. 45 minutes

Preheat oven to 400 F. Wrap steak in plastic wrap, place on a flat surface, and run a rolling pin over to flatten. Take off the wraps. Sprinkle with half of the ricotta cheese, top with spinach, jalapeño pepper, basil, and remaining cheese.

Roll the steak over on the stuffing and secure with toothpicks. Place in a greased baking sheet and cook for 30 minutes, flipping once. Let cool for 3 minutes, slice into pinwheels and serve with sautéed veggies.

Per serving: Cal 490; Net Carbs 2g; Fat 41g; Protein 28g

Prosciutto-Wrapped Chicken with Asparagus

Ingredients for 4 servings

4 chicken breasts
8 prosciutto slices
4 tbsp olive oil
1 lb asparagus spears
2 tbsp fresh lemon juice
Romano cheese for topping

Directions and Total Time: approx. 50 minutes

Preheat oven to 400 F. Season chicken with salt and pepper and wrap 2 prosciutto slices around each chicken breast. Arrange on a lined with parchment paper baking sheet, drizzle with oil, and bake for 25-30 minutes. Preheat grill. Brush asparagus spears with olive oil and grill them for 8-10 minutes, frequently turning until slightly charred. Remove to a plate and drizzle with lemon juice. Grate over Romano cheese and serve with wrapped chicken.

Per serving: Cal 468; Net Carbs 2g; Fat 38g; Protein 26g

Mushroom Broccoli Faux Risotto

Ingredients for 4 servings

1 cup cremini mushrooms, chopped
4 oz butter
2 garlic cloves, minced
1 red onion, finely chopped
1 head broccoli, grated
1 cup water
¾ cup white wine
Salt and black pepper to taste
1 cup coconut cream
¾ cup grated Parmesan
1 tbsp chopped thyme

Directions and Total Time: approx. 25 minutes

Place a pot over medium heat and melt butter. Sauté mushrooms until golden, 5 minutes. Add in garlic and onion and cook for 3 minutes until fragrant and soft.

Mix in broccoli, water, and half of white wine. Season with salt and pepper and simmer for 10 minutes. Mix in coconut cream and simmer until most of the cream evaporates. Turn heat off and stir in Parmesan and thyme. Serve warm.

Per serving: Cal 520; Net Carbs 12g; Fat 43g; Protein 15g

Poultry

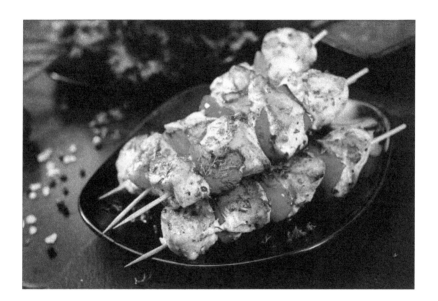

Worcestershire Chicken Peanut Puffs

Ingredients for 4 servings

1 ½ cups chopped chicken thighs, boneless and skinless
1/3 cup peanuts, crushed
1 cup chicken broth
½ cup olive oil
2 tsp Worcestershire sauce
1 tbsp dried parsley
Salt and black pepper to taste
1 tsp celery seeds
¼ tsp cayenne pepper
1 cup almond flour
4 eggs

Directions and Total Time: approx. 30 minutes

In a bowl, combine chicken and peanuts; set aside. In a saucepan over medium heat, mix broth, olive oil, Worcestershire sauce, parsley, salt, pepper, celery seeds, and cayenne pepper. Bring to a boil and stir in almond flour until smooth ball forms. Allow resting for 5 minutes. Add eggs into the batter one after the other and beat until smooth. Mix in chicken and peanuts until well combined. Drop tbsp heaps of the mixture onto a greased baking sheet and bake in the oven at 450 F for 15 minutes. Serve.

Per serving: Cal 514; Net Carbs 1.6g; Fat 47g; Protein 20g

Chargrilled Chili Chicken

Ingredients for 4 servings

3 tbsp chili powder
2 tsp garlic powder
2 tbsp olive oil
1 ½ pounds chicken breasts

Directions and Total Time: approx. 20 minutes

Grease grill grate with cooking spray and preheat to 400 F. Combine chili, salt, black pepper, and garlic in a bowl. Brush chicken with olive oil, sprinkle with the spice mixture and massage with your hands. Grill for 7 minutes per side until well done or to your preference. Serve hot.

Per serving: Cal 253; Net Carbs 1.8g; Fat 15g; Protein 24g

Creamy Chicken with Mushrooms

Ingredients for 4 servings

2 tbsp olive oil
2 garlic cloves, minced
1 onion, sliced into half-moons
1 cup mushrooms, chopped
1 tbsp sweet paprika
1 cup chicken stock
¼ cup dry white wine
1 cup heavy cream
4 chicken breasts, sliced
2 tbsp fresh parsley, chopped

Directions and Total Time: approx. 40 minutes

Heat olive oil in a saucepan and sauté onion and garlic for 3 minutes. Add in chicken and fry for 5 minutes, stirring often. Pour in white wine, mushrooms, and paprika and cook for 4 minutes until the liquid is reduced by half. Pour in the chicken stock. Cook for 20 minutes, stir in heavy cream, and cook for 2 more minutes. Top with parsley.

Per serving: Cal 485; Net Carbs 3.4g; Fat 26g; Protein 57g

Chicken Thighs with Greens

Ingredients for 4 servings

4 chicken thighs
1 cup spinach, chopped
4 green onions, chopped
½ cup Swiss chard, chopped
1 tbsp fresh parsley, chopped
1 cup half-and-half
1 cup vegetable broth
4 tbsp butter

Directions and Total Time: approx. 35 minutes

Melt butter in a skillet and brown the chicken on all sides, about 8 minutes; set aside. Add in green onions and sauté for 2 minutes. Pour in the vegetable broth, return the chicken and bring to a boil. Simmer for 15 minutes. Add in spinach, Swiss chard, and parsley and cook until wilted. Stir in half-and-half for 3-4 minutes. Serve warm.

Per serving: Cal 558; Net Carbs 5.7g; Fat 43g; Protein 35g

Baked Cheese Chicken with Acorn Squash

Ingredients for 6 servings

6 chicken breasts
2 tbsp olive oil
1 lb acorn squash, sliced
Salt and black pepper to taste
1 cup blue cheese, crumbled
2 tbsp parsley, chopped

Directions and Total Time: approx. 45 minutes

Preheat oven to 420 F. Grease a baking dish, add in chicken breasts, salt, pepper, and squash, and drizzle with olive oil. Bake for 20 minutes. Scatter the blue cheese and bake for 15 more minutes. Serve topped with parsley.

Per serving: Cal 235, Net Carbs 5g, Fat 16g, Protein 12g

Chicken & Vegetable Bake

Ingredients for 4 servings

1 lb chicken breasts, sliced
1 tbsp butter
2 green bell peppers, sliced
1 turnip, chopped
1 onion, chopped
1 zucchini, sliced
2 garlic cloves, minced
2 tsp Italian seasoning
Salt and black pepper to taste
8 oz mozzarella, sliced

Directions and Total Time: approx. 45 minutes

Grease a baking dish with cooking spray and place in the chicken slices. Melt butter in a pan over medium heat and sauté onion, zucchini, garlic, bell peppers, turnip, salt, pepper, and Italian seasoning. Cook until tender, 8 minutes. Spread the vegetables over the chicken and cover with cheese slices. Set into the oven and cook until browned for 30 minutes at 370 F. Serve.

Per serving: Cal 341; Net Carbs 8.3g; Fat 13g; Protein 43g

Cheese-Crusted Chicken Breasts

Ingredients for 4 servings

3 tbsp olive oil
3 cups Monterey Jack, grated
2 eggs
½ cup pork rinds, crushed
1 lb chicken breasts, boneless
Salt to taste

Directions and Total Time: approx. 40 minutes

Line a baking sheet with parchment paper. Whisk the eggs with the olive oil in a bowl. Mix the Monterey Jack cheese and pork rinds in another bowl. Season the chicken with salt, dip in egg mixture and coat generously in the cheese mixture. Place on a baking sheet, cover with aluminium foil, and bake in the oven for 25 minutes at 350 F. Remove foil and bake further for 12 minutes until golden brown.

Per serving: Cal 622; Net Carbs 1.2g; Fat 53.8; Protein 45g

Creamy Chicken Thighs with Capers

Ingredients for 4 servings

2 tbsp butter
1 ½ lb chicken thighs
2 cups crème fraîche
8 oz cream cheese
1/3 cup capers
1 tbsp tamari sauce

Directions and Total Time: approx. 30 minutes

Heat oven to 350 F. Melt butter in a skillet and fry the chicken until golden brown, 8 minutes. Transfer to a greased baking sheet, cover with aluminum foil, and bake for 8 minutes. Reserve the butter used to sear the chicken. Remove chicken from the oven, take off the foil, and pour the drippings into a pan along with the butter from frying. Set the chicken aside in a warmer, to serve later. Place the saucepan over low heat and mix in crème fraiche and cream cheese. Simmer until the sauce thickens. Mix in capers and tamari sauce and cook further for 1 minute. Dish the chicken into plates and drizzle the sauce all over.

Per serving: Cal 834; Net Carbs 0.9g; Fat 73g; Protein 36g

Rosemary Chicken& Pumpkin Bake

Ingredients for 4 servings

1 pound chicken thighs
1 pound pumpkin, cubed
½ cup black olives, pitted
3 onion springs, sliced
½ tsp ground cinnamon
¼ tsp ground nutmeg
4 tbsp olive oil
5 garlic cloves, sliced
1 tbsp dried rosemary
Salt and black pepper to taste

Directions and Total Time: approx. 60 minutes

Set oven to 400 F. Place the chicken, skin down in a greased baking dish. Arrange garlic, olives, onions, and pumpkin around the chicken. Drizzle with olive oil. Season with pepper, salt, cinnamon, nutmeg, and rosemary. Bake in the oven for 45 minutes. Serve warm.

Per serving: Cal 431; Net Carbs 6.1g; Fat 34g; Protein 20g

Beef

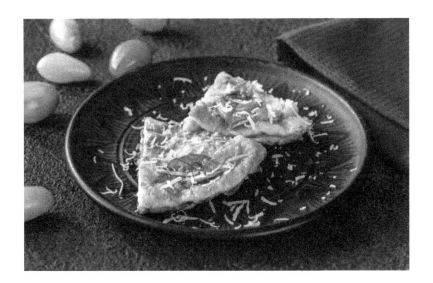

Beef Taco pizza

Ingredients for 4 servings

2 cups shredded mozzarella
2 tbsp cream cheese, softened
1 egg
¾ cup almond flour
1 lb ground beef
2 tsp taco seasoning
½ cup cheese sauce
1 cup grated cheddar cheese
1 cup chopped lettuce
1 tomato, diced
¼ cup sliced black olives
1 cup sour cream for topping

Directions and Total Time: approx. 45 minutes

Preheat oven to 390 F. Line a pizza pan with parchment paper. Microwave the mozzarella and cream cheeses for 1 minute. Remove and mix in egg and almond flour. Spread the mixture on the pan and bake for 15 minutes. Put the beef in a pot and cook for 5 minutes. Stir in taco seasoning. Spread the cheese sauce on the crust and top with the meat. Add cheddar cheese, lettuce, tomato, and black olives. Bake until the cheese melts, 5 minutes. Remove the pizza, drizzle sour cream on top, and serve.

Per serving: Cal 590; Net Carbs 7.9g; Fat 29g; Protein 64g

Beef with Cauli Rice & Cashew Nuts

Ingredients for 4 servings

3 tbsp olive oil
1 ½ lb chuck steak, cubed
2 large eggs, beaten
1 tbsp avocado oil
1 red onion, finely chopped
½ cup chopped bell peppers
½ cup green beans, chopped
3 garlic cloves, minced
4 cups cauliflower rice
¼ cup coconut aminos
1 cup toasted cashew nuts
1 tbsp toasted sesame seeds

Directions and Total Time: approx. 25 minutes

Heat 2 tbsp olive oil in a wok over medium heat and cook the beef until tender, 7-8 minutes; set aside. Pour the eggs in the wok and scramble for 2-3 minutes; set aside. Add the remaining olive oil and avocado oil to heat. Stir in onion, bell peppers, green beans, and garlic. Sauté until soft, 3 minutes. Pour in cauliflower rice, coconut aminos, and stir until evenly combined. Mix in the beef, eggs, and cashew nuts and cook for 3 minutes. Dish into serving plates and garnish with sesame seeds. Serve warm.

Per serving: Cal 500; Net Carbs 3.2g; Fat 32; Protein 44g

Easy Pressure-Cooked Shredded Beef

Ingredients for 4 servings

3 tbsp coconut oil
1 large white onion, chopped
3 garlic cloves, minced
1 cup shredded red cabbage
1 lemon, zested and juiced
1 tsp dried Italian herb blend
1 ½ tbsp balsamic vinegar
½ cup beef broth
2 lb chuck steak
Salt and black pepper to taste

Directions and Total Time: approx. 45 minutes

Select Sauté mode on your pressure cooker. Heat coconut oil and sauté onion, garlic, and red cabbage for 3 minutes. Stir in lemon zest, lemon juice, Italian herb blend, balsamic vinegar, salt, and pepper for 2 minutes; mix in the broth. Place the beef in the cooker. Close the lid, secure the pressure valve, and select Manual/Pressure Cook mode on High for 25 minutes. Once the timer is done, perform a natural pressure release, then a quick pressure release to let out any remaining steam, and open the lid. Remove the beef and using two forks, shred it. Select Sauté and reduce the sauce, 5 minutes. Spoon the pulled beef with sauce over on a bed of zucchini noodles. Serve.

Per serving: Cal 652; Net Carbs 5.8g; Fat 49g; Protein 44g

Mushroom & Bell Pepper Beef Skewers

Ingredients for 4 servings

2 cups cremini mushrooms, halved
2 yellow bell peppers, deseeded and cut into squares
2 lb beef tri-tip steak, cubed
2 tbsp coconut oil
1 tbsp tamari sauce
1 lime, juiced
1 tbsp ginger powder
½ tsp ground cumin

Directions and Total Time: approx. 1 hour 25 minutes

In a bowl, mix coconut oil, tamari sauce, lime juice, ginger, and cumin powder. Add in the beef, mushrooms, and bell peppers; toss to coat. Cover the bowl with a plastic wrap and marinate for 1 hour. Preheat the grill to high heat. Take off the plastic wrap and thread the mushrooms, beef, and bell peppers in this order on skewers until the ingredients are exhausted. Grill the skewers for 5 minutes per side. Remove to serving plates and serve warm with steamed cauliflower rice or braised asparagus.

Per serving: Cal 383; Net Carbs 3.2g; Fat 17g; Protein 51g

Beef & Shiitake Mushroom Stir-Fry

Ingredients for 4 servings

2 cups shiitake mushrooms, halved
2 sprigs rosemary, leaves extracted
1 green bell pepper, chopped
1 lb chuck steak
4 slices prosciutto, chopped
1 tbsp coconut oil
1 tbsp freshly pureed garlic

Directions and Total Time: approx. 30 minutes

Using a sharp knife, slice the chuck steak thinly against the grain and cut into smaller pieces. Heat a skillet over medium heat and cook prosciutto until brown and crispy; set aside. Melt coconut oil in the skillet and cook the beef until brown, 6-8 minutes. Remove to the prosciutto plate. Add mushrooms and bell pepper to the skillet and sauté until softened, 5 minutes. Stir in prosciutto, beef, rosemary, and garlic. Season to taste and cook for 4 minutes. Serve with buttered green beans.

Per serving: Cal 231; Net Carbs 2.1g; Fat 12g; Protein 27g

Coconut Beef with Mushroom & Olive Sauce

Ingredients for 4 servings

¼ cup button mushrooms, sliced
3 tbsp unsalted butter
1 yellow onion, chopped
4 rib-eye steaks
1/3 cup coconut milk
2 tbsp coconut cream
1/2 tsp dried thyme
2 tbsp chopped parsley
3 tbsp black olives, sliced

Directions and Total Time: approx. 30 minutes

Melt 2 tbsp butter in a deep skillet over medium heat. Add and sauté the mushrooms for 4 minutes until tender. Stir in onion and cook further for 3 minutes; set aside. Melt the remaining butter in the skillet and cook the beef for 10 minutes on both sides. Pour mushrooms and onion back to the skillet and add milk, coconut cream, thyme, and 1 tbsp of parsley. Stir and simmer for 2 minutes. Mix in black olives and turn the heat off. Serve garnished with the remaining parsley.

Per serving: Cal 639; Net Carbs 1.9g; Fat 39g; Protein 69g

Maple BBQ Rib Steak

Ingredients for 4 servings

2 lb rib steak, membrane removed
2 tbsp avocado oil
3 tbsp maple syrup, sugar-free
3 tbsp barbecue dry rub

Directions and Total Time: approx. 2 hours 40 minutes

Preheat the oven to 300 F. Line a baking sheet with aluminum foil. In a bowl, mix avocado oil and maple syrup and brush the mixture onto the meat. Sprinkle BBQ rub all over the ribs. Put them in the baking sheet and bake until the meat is tender and crispy on the top, 2 ½ hours. Serve with buttered broccoli and green beans.

Per serving: Cal 490; Net Carbs 1.8g; Fat 26g; Protein 49g

Smoked Paprika Grilled Ribs

Ingredients for 4 servings

4 tbsp sugar-free BBQ sauce + extra for serving
2 tbsp erythritol
Salt and black pepper to taste
1 tbsp olive oil
3 tsp smoked paprika
1 tsp garlic powder
2 lb beef spare ribs

Directions and Total Time: approx. 35 min + chilling time

Mix erythritol, salt, pepper, olive oil, smoked paprika, and garlic powder. Brush on the meaty sides of the ribs and wrap in aluminium foil. Refrigerate for 30 minutes.

Preheat oven to 400 F. Place wrapped ribs on a baking sheet and bake for 40 minutes. Take out the ribs, remove the foil, and brush with BBQ sauce. Brown under the broiler for 4-6 minutes. Serve with extra BBQ sauce.

Per serving: Cal 395; Net Carbs 3g; Fat 33g; Protein 21g

Pork

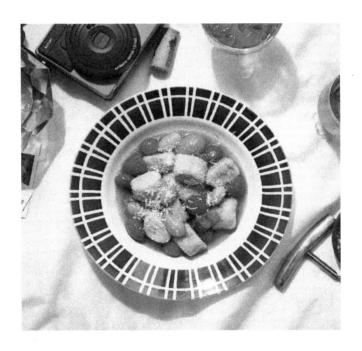

Slow Cooker Pulled Pork

Ingredients for 4 servings

2 tbsp olive oil
½ cup sliced yellow onion
2 lb pork shoulder
4 tbsp taco seasoning
Salt to taste
3 ½ cups chicken broth
5 tbsp psyllium husk powder
1 ¼ cups almond flour
2 eggs, cracked into a bowl
2 tbsp butter

Directions and Total Time: approx. 8 hours 20 minutes

In a skillet, heat olive oil and sauté onion for 3 minutes or until softened. Transfer to the slow cooker. Season pork shoulder with taco seasoning, salt, and place it in the skillet. Sear on each side for 3 minutes and place in the slow cooker. Pour the chicken broth on top. Cover the lid and cook for 7 hours on Low. Shred the pork with two forks. Cook further over low heat for 1 hour; set aside. In a bowl, combine psyllium husk powder, almond flour, and salt. Mix in eggs until a thick dough forms and add 1 cup of water. Separate the dough into 8 pieces.

Lay a parchment paper on a flat surface, grease with cooking spray, and put a dough piece on top. Cover with another parchment paper and, using a rolling pin, flatten the dough into a circle. Repeat the same process for the remaining dough balls. Melt a quarter of the butter in a skillet and cook the flattened dough one after another on both sides until light brown. Transfer the keto tortillas to plates, spoon shredded meat and serve.

Per serving: Cal 520; Net Carbs 3.8g; Fat 30g; Protein 50g

Tasty Pork Chops with Cauliflower Steaks

Ingredients for 4 servings

2 heads cauliflower, cut into 4 steaks
4 pork chops
1 tbsp mesquite seasoning
2 tbsp butter
2 tbsp olive oil
½ cup Parmesan cheese

Directions and Total Time: approx. 30 minutes

Season pork with mesquite flavoring. Melt butter in a skillet and fry pork on both sides for 10 minutes; set aside. Heat olive oil in a grill pan and cook cauli steaks on all sides for 4 minutes. Sprinkle with Parmesan cheese to melt. Serve the pork chops with the cauliflower steaks.

Per serving: Cal 429; Net Carbs 3.9g; Fat 23g; Protein 45g

Lemony Greek Pork Tenderloin

Ingredients for 4 servings

¼ cup olive oil
2 lemon, juiced
2 tbsp Greek seasoning
2 tbsp red wine vinegar
1 ½ lb pork tenderloin
2 tbsp lard

Directions and Total Time: approx. 50 min + chilling time

Preheat oven to 425 F. In a bowl, combine olive oil, lemon juice, Greek seasoning, and red wine vinegar.

Place the pork on a clean flat surface, cut a few incisions, and brush the marinade all over. Cover with plastic wrap and refrigerate for 1 hour. Melt lard in a skillet, remove and unwrap the pork, and sear until brown on the outside. Place in a greased baking dish, brush with any reserved marinade, and bake for 45 minutes. Serve.

Per serving: Cal 383; Net Carbs 2.5g; Fat 24g; Protein 36g

Mushroom Pork Meatballs with Parsnips

Ingredients for 4 servings

1 cup cremini mushrooms, chopped
1 ½ lb ground pork
2 garlic cloves, minced
2 small red onions, chopped
1 tsp dried basil
Salt and black pepper to taste
1 cup grated Parmesan
½ almond milk
2 tbsp olive oil
2 cups tomato sauce
6 fresh basil leaves to garnish
1 lb parsnips, chopped
1 cup water
2 tbsp butter
½ cup coconut cream

Directions and Total Time: approx. 60 minutes

Preheat oven to 350 F. Line a baking tray with parchment paper. In a bowl, add pork, half of the garlic, half of the onion, mushrooms, basil, salt, and pepper and mix until evenly combined. Mold bite-size balls out of the mixture. Pour ½ cup Parmesan cheese and almond milk each in 2 separate bowls. Dip the balls in the milk and then in the cheese. Place on the tray and bake for 20 minutes.

Heat olive oil in a saucepan and sauté the remaining onion and garlic; sauté until fragrant and soft. Pour in tomato sauce and cook for 20 minutes. Add in the meatballs and simmer for 7 minutes. In a pot, add parsnips, 1 cup water, and salt. Bring to a boil and cook for 10 minutes until the parsnips soften. Drain and pour into a bowl. Add butter, salt, and pepper; mash into a puree using a potato mash. Stir in coconut cream and remaining Parmesan cheese until combined. Spoon mashed parsnip into bowls, top with meatballs and sauce, and garnish with basil leaves.

Per serving: Cal 642; Net Carbs 21g; Fat 32g; Protein 50g

Spicy Grilled Pork Spareribs

Ingredients for 4 servings

4 tbsp sugar-free BBQ sauce + extra for serving
2 tbsp erythritol
1 tbsp olive oil
3 tsp cayenne powder
1 tsp garlic powder
1 lb pork spareribs

Directions and Total Time: approx. 60 min + chilling time

Mix erythritol, olive oil, cayenne, and garlic in a bowl. Brush on the meaty sides of the ribs and wrap in foil. Sit for 30 minutes in the fridge. Preheat oven to 400 F, place wrapped ribs on a baking sheet, and cook for 40 minutes. Remove foil, brush with BBQ sauce, and brown under the broiler for 10 minutes on both sides. Serve sliced.

Per serving: Cal 395, Net Carbs 3g, Fat 33g, Protein 21g

Sesame Pork Meatballs

Ingredients for 4 servings

1 lb ground pork
2 scallions, chopped
1 zucchini, grated
4 garlic cloves, minced
1 tsp freshly pureed ginger
1 tsp red chili flakes
2 tbsp tamari sauce
2 tbsp sesame oil
Salt and black pepper to taste
3 tbsp coconut oil

Directions and Total Time: approx. 30 minutes

In a bowl, combine ground pork, scallions, zucchini, garlic, ginger, chili flakes, salt, pepper, tamari sauce, and sesame oil. Form 1-inch oval shapes and place on a plate. Heat coconut oil in a skillet over medium heat and brown the balls for 12 minutes. Transfer to a paper towel-lined plate to drain the excess fat. Serve warm.

Per serving: Cal 296; Net Carbs 1.5g; Fat 22g; Protein 24g

Pork Belly with Creamy Coconut Kale

Ingredients for 4 servings

2 lb pork belly, chopped
Salt and black pepper to taste
2 tbsp coconut oil
1 white onion, chopped
6 cloves garlic, minced
¼ cup ginger thinly sliced
4 long red chilies, halved
1 cup coconut milk
1 cup coconut cream
2 cups chopped kale

Directions and Total Time: approx. 40 min + chilling time

Season pork belly with salt and pepper and refrigerate for 30 minutes. Bring to a boil 2 cups water in a pot, add in pork and cook for 15 minutes. Drain and transfer to a skillet. Warm in half of the coconut oil and fry in the pork for 15 minutes until the skin browns and crackles. Turn a few times to prevent from burning. Spoon onto a plate and discard the fat. Heat the remaining coconut oil in the same skillet and sauté onion, garlic, ginger, and chilies for 5 minutes. Pour in coconut milk and coconut cream and cook for 1 minute. Add kale and cook until wilted, stirring occasionally. Stir in the pork. Cook for 2 minutes. Serve.

Per serving: Cal 608; Net Carbs 6.7g; Fat 36g; Protein 57g

Flavorful Chipotle-Coffee Pork Chops

Ingredients for 4 servings

1 tbsp finely ground coffee
½ tsp chipotle powder
½ tsp garlic powder
Salt and black pepper to taste
½ tsp cumin powder
1 ½ tsp swerve brown sugar
4 bone-in pork chops
2 tbsp lard

Directions and Total Time: approx. 20 min + chilling time

In a bowl, mix coffee, chipotle powder, garlic powder, cumin, salt, pepper, and swerve. Rub spices all over the pork. Cover with plastic wraps and refrigerate overnight. Preheat oven to 350 F. Melt lard in a skillet and sear pork on both sides for 3 minutes. Transfer the skillet to the oven and bake for 10 minutes. Serve with buttered snap peas.

Per serving: Cal 291; Net Carbs 0.5g; Fat 13g; Protein 39g

Seafood

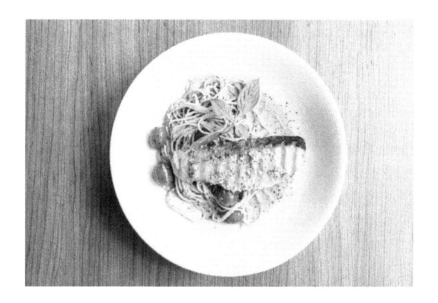

Mahi Mahi with Dill Sour Cream Topping

Ingredients for 4 servings

½ cup grated Pecorino Romano cheese
1 cup sour cream
½ tbsp minced dill
½ lemon, zested and juiced
4 mahi mahi fillets

Directions and Total Time: approx. 30 minutes

Preheat oven to 400 F. Line a baking sheet with parchment paper. In a bowl, mix sour cream, dill, and lemon zest; set aside. Drizzle the mahi mahi with lemon juice and arrange on the baking sheet. Spread sour cream mixture on top and sprinkle with Pecorino Romano cheese. Bake for 15 minutes. Broil the top for 2 minutes until nicely brown. Serve with buttery green beans.

Per serving: Cal 288; Net Carbs 1.2g; Fat 23g; Protein 16g

Mediterranean Tilapia

Ingredients for 4 servings

4 tilapia fillets
2 garlic cloves, minced
½ tsp dry oregano
14 oz canned diced tomatoes
2 tbsp olive oil
½ red onion, chopped
1 tbsp fresh parsley, chopped
¼ cup kalamata olives

Directions and Total Time: approx. 30 minutes

Heat oil in a skillet over medium heat and cook onion for 3 minutes. Add garlic and oregano and cook for 30 seconds.

Stir in tomatoes and bring the mixture to a boil. Reduce the heat and simmer for 5 minutes. Add olives and tilapia. Cook for 8 minutes. Serve topped with parsley.

Per serving: Cal 182; Net Carbs 6g; Fat 15g; Protein 23g

Speedy Tilapia Tacos

Ingredients for 4 servings

1 tbsp olive oil
1 red chili pepper, minced
1 tsp coriander seeds
4 tilapia fillets, chopped
1 tsp smoked paprika
4 low carb tortillas
Salt and black pepper to taste
1 lemon, juiced

Directions and Total Time: approx. 20 minutes

Season the fish with salt, pepper, and paprika. Heat olive oil in a skillet over medium heat. Add tilapia and chili pepper and stir-fry for 6 minutes. Pour in lemon juice and cook for 2 minutes. Divide the fish between the tortillas.

Per serving: Cal 447; Net Carbs 4.3g; Fat 21g; Protein 24g

Cod Fritters with Avocado Salsa

Ingredients for 4 servings

1 lb cod fillets, cubed
¼ cup mayonnaise
¼ cup almond flour
2 eggs
Salt and black pepper to taste
1 cup Swiss cheese, grated
1 tbsp chopped dill
4 tbsp olive oil
1 large avocado, mached
½ cup yogurt
2 tbsp lime juice
2 tbsp fresh cilantro, chopped

Directions and Total Time: approx. 30 minutes

In a bowl, mix the cod cubes, mayonnaise, flour, eggs, salt, pepper, Swiss cheese, and dill. Warm 2 tbsp of olive oil in a skillet over medium heat. Fetch 2 tbsp of the fish mixture into the skillet and use the back of a spatula to flatten the top. Cook for 4 minutes, flip, and fry for 4 more minutes. Remove onto a wire rack and repeat until the fish batter is over. In a small bowl, mix the avocado, lime juice, yogurt, cilantro, salt, and pepper. Serve with the fritters.

Per serving: Cal 633; Net Carbs 7g; Fat 46.9g; Protein 39g

Vegan and vegetarian

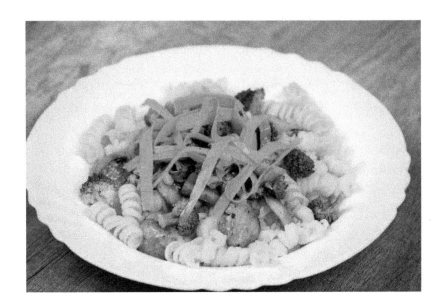

Stuffed Portobello Mushrooms

Ingredients for 2 servings

4 Portobello mushrooms
2 tbsp olive oil
2 cups lettuce
1 cup crumbled blue cheese

Directions and Total Time: approx. 30 minutes

Preheat oven to 350 F. Remove the stems from the mushrooms. Fill the mushrooms with blue cheese and place on a lined baking sheet. Bake for about 20 minutes. Serve with lettuce drizzled with olive oil.

Per serving: Cal 334; Net Carbs 5.5g; Fat 29g; Protein 14g

Cheesy Roasted Vegetable Spaghetti

Ingredients for 4 servings

2 (8 oz) packs shirataki spaghetti
1 cup chopped mixed bell peppers
½ cup grated Parmesan cheese for topping
1 lb asparagus, chopped
1 cup broccoli florets
1 cup green beans, chopped
3 tbsp olive oil
1 small onion, chopped
2 garlic cloves, minced
1 cup diced tomatoes
½ cup chopped basil

Directions and Total Time: approx. 45 minutes

Boil 2 cups water in a pot. Strain the shirataki pasta and rinse well under hot running water. Allow draining and pour the shirataki pasta into the boiling water. Cook for 3 minutes and strain again. Place a dry skillet and stir-fry the shirataki pasta until visibly dry, 1-2 minutes; set aside. Preheat oven to 425 F. In a bowl, add asparagus, broccoli, bell peppers, and green beans and toss with half of olive oil. Spread the vegetables on a baking sheet and roast for 20 minutes. Heat the remaining olive oil in a skillet and sauté onion and garlic for 3 minutes. Stir in tomatoes and cook for 8 minutes. Mix in shirataki and vegetables. Top with Parmesan cheese and serve.

Per serving: Cal 272; Net Carbs 7g; Fats 12g; Protein 12g

Vegetarian Ketogenic Burgers

Ingredients for 2 servings

1 garlic cloves, minced
2 Portobello mushrooms
1 tbsp coconut oil, melted
1 tbsp chopped basil
1 tbsp oregano
2 eggs, fried
2 zero carb buns
2 tbsp mayonnaise
2 lettuce leaves
Salt to taste

Directions and Total Time: approx. 20 minutes

Combine the coconut oil, garlic, basil, oregano, and salt in a bowl. Place the mushrooms in the bowl and coat well. Preheat the grill to medium. Grill the mushrooms about 2 minutes per side. Slice them and grill for 2 minutes per side. Cut the buns in half. Add the lettuce leaves, mushrooms, eggs, and mayo. Top with the other bun.

Per serving: Cal 637; Net Carbs 8.5g; Fat 53g; Protein 23g

Tempeh Taco Cups

Ingredients for 4 servings

8 iceberg lettuce leaves
4 zero carb tortilla wraps
2 tsp melted butter
1 tbsp olive oil
1 yellow onion, chopped
½ cup tempeh, crumbled
1 tsp smoked paprika
½ tsp cumin powder
1 red bell pepper, chopped
1 avocado, halved and pitted
1 small lemon, juiced
¼ cup sour cream

Directions and Total Time: approx. 30 minutes

Preheat oven to 400 F. Divide each tortilla wrap into 2, lay on a chopping board, and brush with butter. Line 8 muffin tins with the tortilla and bake for 9 minutes.

Heat olive oil in a skillet and sauté onion for 3 minutes. Crumble tempeh into the pan and cook for 8 minutes. Stir in paprika and cumin and cook for 1 minute. To assemble, fit lettuce leaves into the tortilla cups, share tempeh mixture on top, top with bell pepper, avocado, and drizzle with lemon juice. Add sour cream and serve.

Per serving: Cal 220; Net Carbs 3.8g, Fat 17g, Protein 6.7g

Rich Veggie Pasta Primavera

Ingredients for 4 servings

2 cups cauliflower florets, cut into matchsticks
½ cup grated Pecorino Romano cheese
1 cup shredded mozzarella
½ cup chopped green onions
1 egg yolk
¼ cup olive oil
1 cup spring onions, sliced
4 garlic cloves, minced
1 cup grape tomatoes, halved
2 tsp dried Italian seasoning
½ lemon, juiced
2 tbsp chopped fresh parsley

Directions and Total Time: approx. 25 min + chilling time

Microwave mozzarella cheese for 2 minutes. Take out the bowl and let cool for 1 minute. Mix in egg yolk until well-combined. Lay a parchment paper on a flat surface, pour the cheese mixture on top and cover with another parchment paper. Flatten the dough into 1/8-inch thickness. Take off the parchment paper and cut the dough into penne-size pieces. Place in a bowl and refrigerate overnight. Bring 2 cups water to a boil and add in penne. Cook for 1 minute and drain; set aside. Heat olive oil in a skillet and sauté onion, garlic, cauliflower, and spring onions for 7 minutes. Stir in tomatoes and Italian seasoning and cook for 5 minutes. Mix in lemon juice and penne. Top with Pecorino Romano cheese and serve.

Per serving: Cal 283; Net Carbs 5g; Fats 18g; Protein 15g

Mushroom White Pizza

Ingredients for 4 servings

2 eggs
½ cup mayonnaise
¾ cup almond flour
1 tbsp psyllium husk powder
1 tsp baking soda
½ tsp salt
¼ cup mushrooms, sliced
1 tbsp oregano
1 tbsp basil pesto
2 tbsp olive oil
Salt and black pepper to taste
½ cup coconut cream
¾ cup Parmesan, shredded
6 black olives

Directions and Total Time: approx. 35 minutes

In a bowl, whisk eggs and mix in mayonnaise, almond flour, psyllium husk powder, baking soda, and salt. Allow sitting for 5 minutes. Pour the batter into a greased baking sheet. Bake for 10 minutes at 350 F. In a bowl, mix mushrooms with pesto, olive oil, salt, and pepper. Remove the crust from the oven and spread the coconut cream on top. Add the mushroom mixture and Parmesan cheese. Bake the pizza further until the cheese melts, about 10 minutes. Spread the olives on top and serve.

Per serving: Cal 346; Net Carbs 5.5g; Fat 32.7g; Protein 8g

Cheesy Broccoli Nachos with Salsa

Ingredients for 4 servings

2 heads broccoli, chopped
3 tbsp coconut flour
1 tsp smoked paprika
½ tsp coriander powder
1 tsp cumin powder
½ tsp garlic powder
2 eggs, beaten
¼ cup grated Monterey Jack
4 plum tomatoes, chopped
½ lime, juiced
4 sprigs cilantro, chopped
1 avocado, chopped

Directions and Total Time: approx. 30 minutes

Preheat oven to 350 F. Pour broccoli in a food processor and blend into a rice-like consistency. Heat a skillet over low heat, pour in broccoli, and fry for 10 minutes. Transfer to a bowl. Line 2 baking sheets with parchment papers. To the broccoli, add coconut flour, paprika, coriander powder, cumin, garlic, and eggs. Mix and form into a ball. Divide into halves, place each half on each baking sheet, and press down into a rough circle. Bake for 10 minutes. Take out of the oven, cut into triangles, and sprinkle with Monterey Jack cheese; let cool. In a bowl, combine tomatoes, lime, cilantro, and avocado. Serve nachos with salsa.

Per serving: Cal 208; Net Carbs 4.5g, Fat 12.4g, Protein 7g

Snacks and side dish

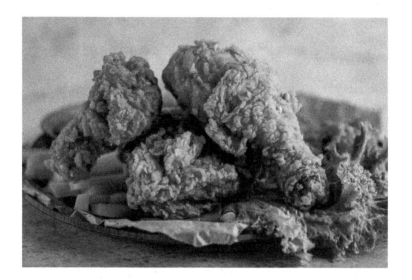

Chili Baked Zucchini Sticks with Aioli

Ingredients for 4 servings

¼ cup Pecorino Romano cheese, shredded
¼ cup pork rind crumbs
1 tsp sweet paprika
Salt and chili pepper to taste
1 cup mayonnaise
Juice from half lemon
2 garlic cloves, minced
3 fresh eggs
2 zucchinis, cut into strips

Directions and Total Time: approx. 25 minutes

Preheat oven to 425 F. Line a baking sheet with foil. In a bowl, mix pork rinds, paprika, Pecorino Romano cheese, salt, and chili pepper. Beat the eggs in another bowl. Coat zucchini strips in eggs, then in the cheese mixture, and arrange on the sheet. Grease lightly with cooking spray and bake for 15 minutes. Combine in a bowl mayonnaise, lemon juice, and garlic, and gently stir until everything is well incorporated. Serve the strips with aioli.

Per serving: Cal 180; Net Carbs 2g; Fat 14g; Protein 6g

Cauliflower Rice & Bacon Gratin

Ingredients for 4 servings

1 cup canned artichoke hearts, drained and chopped
6 bacon slices, chopped
2 cups cauliflower rice
3 cups baby spinach, chopped
1 garlic clove, minced
1 tbsp olive oil
Salt and black pepper to taste
¼ cup sour cream
8 oz cream cheese, softened
¼ cup grated Parmesan
1 ½ cups grated mozzarella

Directions and Total Time: approx. 30 minutes

Preheat oven to 350 F. Cook bacon in a skillet over medium heat until brown and crispy, 5 minutes. Spoon onto a plate. In a bowl, mix cauli rice, artichokes, spinach, garlic, olive oil, salt, pepper, sour cream, cream cheese, bacon, and half of Parmesan cheese. Spread the mixture onto a baking dish and top with the remaining Parmesan and mozzarella cheeses. Bake for 15 minutes. Serve.

Per serving: Cal 500; Net Carbs 5.3g; Fat 37g; Protein 28g

Delicious Pancetta Strawberries

Ingredients for 4 servings

2 tbsp swerve confectioner's sugar
1 cup mascarpone cheese
1/8 tsp white pepper
12 fresh strawberries
12 thin slices pancetta

Directions and Total Time: approx. 30 minutes

In a bowl, combine mascarpone, swerve confectioner's sugar, and white pepper. Coat strawberries in the mixture, wrap each strawberry in a pancetta slice, and place on an ungreased baking sheet. Bake in the oven at 425 F for 15-20 minutes until pancetta browns. Serve warm.

Per serving: Cal 171; Net Carbs 1.2g; Fat 11g; Protein 12g

Creamy Ham & Parsnip Puree

Ingredients for 4 servings

1 lb parsnips, diced
3 tbsp olive oil, divided
2 tsp garlic powder
¾ cup almond milk
4 tbsp heavy cream
4 tbsp butter
6 slices deli ham, chopped
2 tsp freshly chopped oregano

Directions and Total Time: approx. 45 minutes

Preheat oven to 400 F. Spread parsnips on a baking sheet and drizzle with 2 tbsp olive oil. Cover tightly with aluminum foil and bake until the parsnips are tender, 40 minutes. Remove from the oven, take off the foil, and transfer to a bowl. Add in garlic powder, almond milk, heavy cream, and butter. With an immersion blender, puree the ingredients until smooth. Fold in the ham and sprinkle with oregano. Serve.

Per serving: Cal 477; Net Carbs 20g; Fat 30g; Protein 10g

Roasted Ham with Radishes

Ingredients for 4 servings

1 lb radishes, halved
Salt and black pepper to taste
1 tbsp butter, melted
3 slices deli ham, chopped

Directions and Total Time: approx. 30 minutes

Preheat oven to 375 F. Arrange the radishes on a greased baking sheet. Season with salt and pepper and sprinkle with butter and ham. Bake for 25 minutes. Serve warm.

Per serving: Cal 68; Net Carbs 0.5g; Fat 4g; Protein 4g

Rosemary Cheese Chips with Guacamole

Ingredients for 4 servings

1 tbsp rosemary, chopped
1 cup Grana Padano, grated
¼ tsp sweet paprika
¼ tsp garlic powder
2 avocados, pitted and scooped
1 tomato, chopped

Directions and Total Time: approx. 20 minutes

Preheat oven to 350 F. Line a baking sheet with parchment paper. Mix Grana Padano cheese, paprika, rosemary, and garlic powder evenly. Spoon 6-8 teaspoons on the baking sheet creating spaces between each mound; flatten mounds. Bake for 5 minutes, cool, and remove to a plate. To make the guacamole, mash avocados with a fork in a bowl, add in tomato, and continue to mash until mostly smooth; season. Serve chips with guacamole.

Per serving: Cal 229; Net Carbs 2g; Fat 20g; Protein 10g

Chive & Green Bean Ham Rolls

Ingredients for 4 servings

8 oz Havarti cheese, cut into 16 strips
16 thin slices deli ham, cut in half lengthwise
1 medium sweet red pepper, cut into 16 strips
1 ½ cups water
16 fresh green beans
2 tbsp salted butter
16 whole chives

Directions and Total Time: approx. 15 min + chilling time

Bring the water to a boil in a saucepan over medium heat. Add in green beans, cover, and cook for 3 minutes or until softened; drain. Melt butter in a skillet and sauté green beans for 2 minutes; transfer to a plate. Assemble 1 green bean, 1 strip of red pepper, 1 cheese strip, and wrap with a ham slice. Tie with one chive. Repeat the assembling process with the remaining ingredients and refrigerate.

Per serving: Cal 399; Net Carbs 8.7g; Fat 24g; Protein 35g

Dessert

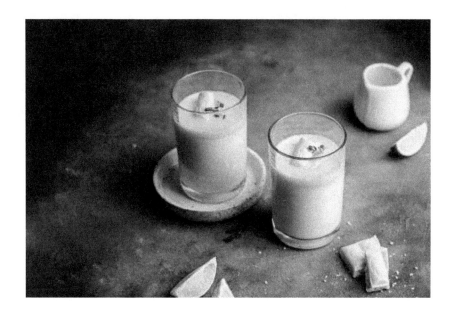

Coconut Butter Ice Cream

Ingredients for 4 servings

½ cup smooth coconut butter
½ cup swerve sugar
3 cups half and half
1 tsp vanilla extract

Directions and Total Time: approx. 10 min + freezing time

Beat coconut butter and swerve sugar in a bowl with a hand mixer until smooth. Gradually whisk in half and half until thoroughly combined. Mix in vanilla. Pour the mixture into a loaf pan and freeze for 45 minutes until firmed up. Scoop into glasses when ready to eat and serve.

Per serving: Cal 290; Net Carbs 6g; Fat 23g; Protein 13g

Chia Pudding

Ingredients for 4 servings

4 tbsp chia seeds
½ cup almond milk
1 cup coconut cream
½ cup sour cream
½ tsp vanilla extract
¼ tsp cardamon powder
1 tbsp stevia

Directions and Total Time: approx. 20 min + cooling time

Add all the ingredients in a mixing bowl and stir to combine. Leave to rest for 20 minutes. Apportion the mixture among bowls. Serve and enjoy!

Per serving: Cal 258; Net Carbs: 2g; Fat: 24g; Protein: 5g

Mom's Walnut Cookies

Ingredients for 12 servings

1 egg
2 cups ground pecans
¼ cup sweetener
½ tsp baking soda
1 tbsp ghee
20 walnuts, chopped

Directions and Total Time: approx. 25 minutes

Preheat oven to 350 F. In a bowl, mix all the ingredients, except for walnuts, until combined. Make balls out of the mixture and press them with your thumb onto a lined cookie sheet. Top with walnuts. Bake for 12 minutes.

Per serving: Cal 101; Net Carbs: 1g; Fat: 11g; Protein: 2g

Almond Ice Cream

Ingredients for 4 servings

2 cups heavy cream
1 tbsp xylitol
½ cup smooth almond butter
1 tbsp olive oil
1 tbsp vanilla extract
½ tsp salt
2 egg yolks
½ cup almonds, chopped

½ cup swerve sugar

Directions and Total Time: approx. 40 min + cooling time

Warm heavy cream with almond butter, olive oil, xylitol, and salt in a small pan over low heat without boiling, for 3 minutes. Beat the egg yolks until creamy in color. Stir the eggs into the cream mixture. Refrigerate cream mixture for 30 minutes. Remove and stir in swerve sugar. Pour mixture into ice cream machine and churn it according to the manufacturer's instructions. Stir in almonds and spoon mixture into loaf pan. Refrigerate for at least for 2 hours.

Per serving: Cal 552; Net Carbs 6.2g; Fat 45.4g; Protein 9g

Dark Chocolate Cheesecake Bites

Ingredients for 6 servings

10 oz unsweetened dark chocolate chips
½ cup half and half
20 oz cream cheese, softened
½ cup swerve sugar
1 tsp vanilla extract

Directions and Total Time: approx. 5 min + cooling time

In a saucepan, melt the chocolate with half and a half over low heat for 1 minute. Turn the heat off. In a bowl, whisk the cream cheese, swerve sugar, and vanilla with a hand mixer until smooth. Stir into the chocolate mixture. Spoon into silicone muffin tins and freeze for 4 hours until firm.

Per serving: Cal 241; Net Carbs 3.1g; Fat 22g; Protein 5g

Cardamom Cookies

Ingredients for 4 servings

2 cups almond flour
½ tsp baking soda
¾ cup sweetener
½ cup butter, softened
1 tbsp vanilla extract

Coating:
2 tbsp erythritol
1 tsp ground cardamom

Directions and Total Time: approx. 25 minutes

Preheat your oven to 350 F. Combine all cookie ingredients in a bowl. Make balls out of the mixture and flatten them with hands. Combine the cardamom and erythritol. Dip the cookies in the cardamom mixture and arrange them on a lined cookie sheet. Cook for 15 minutes until crispy.

Per serving: Cal 131; Net Carbs: 1g; Fat: 13g; Protein: 3g

Chocolate Ice Bombs

Ingredients for 4 servings

2 tbsp butter, melted
1 cup mascarpone cheese
4 tbsp xylitol
1 tbsp dark rum
2 tbsp cocoa powder
2 ½ oz dark chocolate, melted

Directions and Total Time: approx. 10 min + cooling time

Blitz mascarpone cheese, xylitol, rum, and cocoa powder, in a food processor until mixed. Roll 2 tbsp of the mixture and place on a lined tray. Mix melted butter and chocolate, and coat the bombs with it. Freeze for 2 hours.

Per serving: Cal 286; Net Carbs 7.2g; Fat 23g; Protein 10

CPSIA information can be obtained
at www.ICGtesting.com
Printed in the USA
BVHW051353080321
601998BV00011BA/1321